Ten Important Things You Should Know About Life

Book #2

—

Stress and Stress-Related Illnesses

By

Allen Lawrence, M.D., Ph.D.
Lisa Robyn Lawrence, M.S., Ph.D.

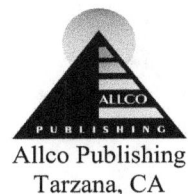

Allco Publishing
Tarzana, CA

Copyright © 2015 by Allen Lawrence, M.D. & Lisa Robyn Lawrence, M.S., Ph.D.

Ten Important Things You Should Know About Life – Stress and Stress-Related Illnesses

Price $ 9.95

All rights reserved. No part of this book may be reproduced or transmitted in any form or by any means, electronic or mechanical, including photocopying, recording, or by any information storage or retrieval system without permission in writing from the publisher, except for the inclusion of quotations in a review. Requests for such permissions should be addressed to ALLCO Publishing.

This book is a reference work based on research by the authors.
The directions stated in this book are in no way to be considered as a substitute for consultation or appropriate treatment by a duly licensed physician.

Printed in the United States of America

ALLCO Publishing
18653 Ventura Blvd., #384
Tarzana, CA 91356

Info@AllcoPublishing.com

ACKNOWLEDGMENTS

The books in this series could not be possible without many years of seeking and searching for information, knowledge, wisdom and the truth. We have many people to thank for our understandings of the nature of life, the universe and the insights we have achieved here in and in our lives.

I offer thanks to the many men and women who have sacrificed their health and well-being to the medical profession. Most thought that what they were doing was right, that medical doctors and the medical system could cure them or at least help them heal themselves. This unfortunately does not always happen, and in many cases, many people have suffered much more than they should have. This is unfortunate and our goal here is to stop this from happening.

We dedicate this book to these people and to all of those people who yet will end up with the same fate. We hope that these books along with our other books can help prevent and protect you from a system which is unable to give you the positive results you desire, the healing and curing of your illnesses. It is our mission to help individuals when the medical system can't, please read and learn how to help yourself.

We would like to offer special notice to two very good friend of ours, Mason Rose, III and his wife, Marlene Rose, from who we learned a great deal in our seeking journeys. Mason asked us questions and forced us to think, look and understand. Thank you, Mason and Marlene.

Many thanks to Mom Sally for she was always an inspiration.

In no specific order special thanks to: Itzthak Bentov, Stanislav Grof, M.D., Louise Hay, Ken Keyes, M. Scott Peck, M.D., Maxwell Maltz, M.D., Richard Bach, Fritjof Capra, Ph.D. and so many others as it would be impossible to list them all.

PROLOGUE

To my knowledge no person is born and handed a manual to help them either understand or make life work for them so that they can have all that life has to offer. While we would love to write such a manual, and we have tried, the amount of material that would be needed to be complete and tell what needed to be told, would literally be astronomical. It would, we believe, end up being a task that could literally take a life time. Instead, we asked our self if there were at least 10 most important points or things everyone should know about life. Ten points that could help us each make our life work a little better for us, individually, as a couple and as a family. We know life is difficult but we also know that there is information that can make life easier and more productive. This is how and why we started this project and, if you are reading this, this what we ended up with a series of short readable books that can help everyone better understand life and how to make it work for them.

For most people it is not entirely easy to fully understand what life is nor how to make life work for them. If we cannot fully understand what life is and how we can make it works for us, how can we really get the very best out of our life? How can we help our loved ones, family and friends make it work for them. How can we really know and understand what is really most dear in our life? While some people do find ways to get close to understanding, most are literally millions of miles away. If, however, some of us are able to make life work for us, then we believe it can then be possible for everyone, if they have the right information, to make life work for them.

Here are 10 points of information about stress and stress-related illnesses which can help you create a huge difference in for your life, allowing you to live the life you want, rather than the life you are dealt. Your overall quality of life, your life experience, your health, your overall well-being are actually based on these 10 points of information and whether you can make them work for you or against you. If you use them correctly, then you will benefit. If you ignore or avoid them, then your life will be harder and more likely problematic.

In a sense these 10 points about stress and stress-related illnesses make up the rules and operating principles upon which we as human beings live our life, as well as whether we live our life fully or only partially. Using these 10 points about stress and stress-related illness appropriately allows us to be productive, and to create and maintain optimal physical, mental, emotional and spiritual health and wellness.

These 10 principles operate everywhere in our world and possibly everywhere in the Universe simultaneously. They operate regardless of where you go (at least on planet Earth), no matter what you are doing, nor who you are. They operate 24-7-365, for as long as our Universe exists. They are the backbone of humanity and the foundation of human life.

We offer these *10 Things You Should Know About Life – Stress And Stress-Related Illnesses* to everyone everywhere, but we also realize that to fully understand these 10 Points will have to have reached a level of insight that puts you on the path to enlightenment and wisdom. While understanding the words that define them is important, understanding their underlying message, the message offered below the level of the words, is more important. Read the words but think about and work on their meaning and what doors they will open for you as you move forward in life toward full evolution, enlightenment and wisdom.

FOREWORD

If you are reading this book then it is likely that you are alive and sentient. It is also likely that you are a "Seeker" or "Searcher," someone who is looking for answers and trying to understand not just the world you live in, but life itself. One important quality searchers must have is that they must ask questions. They must ask questions not just because they are seeking answers to important questions, but because the answers they seek are not commonly understood by the average person. The questions themselves and their answers are often as old as humanity itself. In this work, *10 Things You Should Know About Life – Stress And Stress-Related Illness*es, we offer some basic answers to age old questions regarding how illness is created and what you can do about it. These answers once understood will then offer other answers regarding who we are, what life is about, how stress affects us, where illness comes from and how you can make sense of what is happening to you and others in the world around you.

As we see it, the answers to all questions about life are always right in front of us. They are everywhere. They are part of life itself. They are reflected in both the material and spiritual universes as the Intelligent Universe we live in has been constructed to give us all the answers we need to make life work for us. Life allows us to ask questions, seek the truth and find it. We believe that the answer to any and every question you have or will ask about life are always right in front of you, in plain sight. While we may not think or believe that we can see, hear, feel and/or experience them, they are still always right there ready and waiting for us. All we have to do is "know" that they are the answers we seek, when we see, hear, feel or experience them.

We ask you now to "open your eyes and see." To see what life is really about. On one level, our human level, we are essentially blind for we see only situations, events and physical activities, the movements and actions of life. When we see only in this way, as a mortal human being, we see life as a series of events that may take place either directly in front of us, or in print, on a screen, as with movies and TV or as text. While there are emotions involved we often have no immediate idea as to what has happened before the moment we are living or what will occur because of these events in the future. We are often not entirely connected to full meaning or understanding of what is really happening. Even when we are directly involved, the most we can generally consider is the story about what we see and what we believe is happening in the now moment.

We can, when we open our physical eyes, look around at our surroundings and we see all that is in our physical view and nothing more. This is what most people believe life is all about, what they see, what they feel and what they touch. This is what happens at our higher animal level, where we take physical energy of light waves and using these physical energies we see people and events, what is happening to people and how they are affected by these events and situations, merely as impresses and motion, positive or negative action. We are primarily only interested in whether they are threatening or non-threatening, whether we are in danger or not. We see who and what is in the room, but we are not interested in what they are doing nor who they are or what they are doing, only whether they are friends or enemies. Whether they are treats or not.

At our higher human levels do we of course care about what they are actually doing (other than only through our curiosity), as well as who they are as people. We may even be interested in what they are not doing as we are more aware of the world and how it works. At the human level threat is also important but we are often more interested in information, reasons and we can look below physical appearances to see essences. We can look at people and situations to see underlying meanings and so that we can "really know" what is going on.

On still another level, a level we might think of as our Higher Self level, when we open our eyes, we are opening our spiritual eyes and see even more of what is really around us. We see who everyone is spiritually and how they fit into our spiritual nature of life. We can now recognize spiritual actions, purposes, goals and truths.

When we understand and use all three of our levels our lower self or animal level, our middle self or human level, and our Higher Self or spiritual level, we now have a real understanding of what life is and who we are. Most days however, we only use our first two levels, our lower self and middle self levels and hence we only know part, often only a very, very small part of who we are and what life is really about.

In this work we will ask you to go past your lower self, animal level, and past your middle self, human level and read our words, listen to them not just with your head, heart and conscious mind, but to try to make sense of them on all three of our levels, the physical level of energy, action and time, read and see what we offer also on your human level understanding, and also see, read, hear, feel and listen the our underlying messages and meanings, what we are trying to tell you about life and what is important about making your life work for you, also with your Higher Self level as well.

We now want to offer you a deeper understanding that what goes on in your "real" life and within the Intelligent Universe around you and how everything ultimately affects you. We now ask you to recognize that what you see, feel and hear on your human level and who you interpret this information through your Higher Self level, can allow you to make much more sense and meaning of your life, of yourself and in your "real"place in life.

Finally, we ask you to open your physical eyes and see exactly what is really going on around you and how you can change your beliefs and actions and in doing so reduce and/or entirely eliminate stress and stress-related illnesses. We ask you to understand that there are aspects of life that exist on more than just the physical levels of atoms, molecules, chemical compounds, energy, light waves, sound waves and physical impresses and human events. That our world, that the Intelligent Universe you live in, is much greater than you now can ever understand it to be. That there a re many dimensions and that there are not only a human aspects to it, and that your living in this

Intelligent Universe is no accident but has a higher and even more important purpose. We ask you to recognize and learn that no matter where you live, where you go, all that you see in the physical world has been created by humans for humans and was ultimately created for us human beings by our Higher Self and the Intelligent Universe we live in, upon our request in order to supports us, nourish us, act as our protector, be our teacher, our parent, our child, our enemy and our friend, so that we live 100% in life, but also live fully within the spiritual yet physical universe. When you understand all of this fully, then, and only then, will you be able to fully relate to 1) our otherwise unfathomable depths of your humanity, and 2) the otherwise unfathomable depths of our Intelligent Universe.

We will also herein offer you a new, different and more evolved view of standard Western medicine and the world of dealing with, preventing and managing illness, and especially those illnesses and Stress-Related Disorder caused by or made worse by stress. That is, we will offer you the ability to find and understand the real and true meaning and intention of illness as opposed to your "blind" interpretation of what you and the medical profession think or believe illness really is. Once you truly understand what illness is about then you will be able to better deal with, treat, eliminate and evolve yourself from the illnesses you have and those you prevent to an individual who never has to be ill, ever again.

As you understands more about stress and stress-related illnesses you will recognize that you already knew a great deal about how you have become ill in the past and because of what you now know, you will soon begin to shed new light upon your life and your well-being. Through this new way of thinking and seeing the world, your health, and the Western medical profession, you will become enlightened and you will now have information to heal and protect yourself from future illnesses, disability and premature death. As you find these new answers, you will also find that they have always been there right in front of you, right in front of your eyes. All that you now have to do is open your eyes, see the truth, move forward, evolve and reach a stage in life where you can, on our own or with help, see the truth of yourself and your life.

We hope that this work will help you to open your eyes and see a bright and more evolved picture of who you are, what life is really about and then while doing so, find and accept both enlightenment and wisdom.

TABLE OF CONTENTS

Acknowledgments. iii
Prologue. iv
Forward. vi

One –   The Definition And Scope of Stress. 1
Two –   Stress And The Laws Of Our Intelligent Universe. 7
Three –   Negative "Bad" Stress Verus Positive "Good" Stress. . . 9
Four –   Stress and Illness. 15
Five –   Stress Chronic Disease, Disability and Premature
          Death. 19
Six –   Stress Is an Intelligent Act of Your Body and
          Body-Mind. 23
Seven –   Stress Is a Teacher - Stress Can Lead to Learning,
          Growth, Evolution and Wisdom. 27
Eight –   Stress and Solving Unresolved Conflicts. 31
Nine –   Eliminating Stress - Challenges and Opportunities. . . . 35
Ten –   Avoid Treating Stress Medically. 37

Epilogue. 43

End Notes. 47

ONE

THE DEFINITION AND SCOPE OF STRESS

Stress has been defined in many different ways. In this book we plan to offer a simple, yet potent, definition of stress, one which we believe can help you, understand what stress is and how it can effect you. Before we present our definition we want to present at least one very common dictionary definition of stress so that you can contrast this standard definition of stress with our definition of stress. We are doing this to demonstrate how difficult it is to really understand stress from what is available to the generally public. One of the more common dictionary definitions of stress tell us only that stress is: "A state of mental, emotional, or other strain. Another definition tells us that stress is: "Subject to pressure, tension, or strain." Stress has also been defined and explained as series of anatomical and physiologic actions and reactions that are designed to protect an individual from injury or death. While all of these definitions are accurate definition, they do not always help us really understand exactly what stress is nor how to manage stress, nor how it can or will affect you as an individual.

In order to answer these question and be more precise we off er what we believe is more practical definition of stress, "Stress is the difference between the way we want our life or world to be and the way it actually is." An even simpler definition is, "Stress is created when there is a difference between what you want and what you get. The greater difference between what you have and what you want, the greater the degree of stress."

While the first dictionary definition explains stress as a set of symptoms and signs, our definitions tries to bring stress to us as a human issue. Stress is not what happens to you, but instead how we see the world and/or our life, here stress is created based on how we individually perceive our life and how we perceive the word around us. Stress occurs because we are threatened by what we want or don't want, what we have and what we don't have, and how these then affect us, because of what we want, think or choose to believe. Stress occurs not from what is outside of us but from how we think and what we believe, from what is going on within us.

In other words, stress is not created out side of us by what is happening or not happening, but rater from within by what we want or don't want in our life.

> Stress Is the Difference Between
> The Way We Want Your World to Be
> And the Way it Actually Is.

The Stress Mechanism itself is an ancient internal system that is present in virtually every known form of life on planet Earth. Whether in a one-celled creature or a human being, the Stress Mechanism exists in order to protect all life forms and allow them to either move away from danger or to attack anything that threatens us, so that we can protect ourselves. Whether what the organism perceives is true or false, whether the threat is real or imagined, whether the other organism or situation might or definitely will cause harm, injury or death, is ultimately less important than that we perceive that it might and that we do something, act, to protect ourselves, before we are destroyed.

The Stress Mechanism, which also commonly referred to as the Fight or Flight Mechanism, is made up of multiple body systems, each of which are designed to react instantly so that the individual does not have to think, but instead merely react, to any and all potential life threatening dangers.

Because of the stress mechanism we react to any and all situations, events, potential, imagining or real threats, by triggering and activating the Stress Mechanisms even before we have had time to think about or decide what to do. These things, situations, events, or threats, which trigger and activate of the stress mechanism are commonly called *Stressors*. In reality our stress reaction is not actually triggered directly or physically by these stressors, but rather by our perception that we are being threatened, that there is a real, or imagined, threat to our life and to our overall well-being.

Stress therefore is a perceived event, one which we can control and train ourselves out of. For example police officers, fire fighters, doctors, race drivers and a host of other people who are at times threatened by either potential or actual threatening events or situations, generally learn how not to become stressed by work threats so that they can do their jobs correctly and effectively.

While these events, situations or things can and often do create extreme stress reactions in the general public, those who are trained to deal with them either have no stress or very little stress when confronted by these stressors. This means that we, you and I, as well as the general public, can also train ourselves out of being stressed by virtually any and all situations. This also means, that with a little forethought, and if needed some training, we can learn to rapidly manage or eliminate stress so that we reduce all of the potential negative affects of stress that might affects us if we allowed ourselves to be chronically stressed.

Positive and Negative Stress

Generally when most people think about stress they think about the negative aspects of stress, and hence about negative stress. Stress however, can actually be either positive and negative. That is, stress can trigger a sense of threat, fear, anxiety, discomfort, lot of physical, mental and emotional responses, and when left unresolved, chronic or recurrent stress can undermine and sabotage your body, but it can also trigger good feelings and a positive experience. When negative stress is potentially bad for you, positive stress can actually be good for you. It can help you to improve your health and even heal many types of illnesses.

Acute and Chronic Stress

Stress can either be in the form of acute or chronic stress. Acute stress means that whatever is taking place is taking place right now and the stress being experienced is occurring from what is happening in the moment. The events and stress created generally have a sharp onset and a relatively well defined end point. Chronic stress implies that whatever is causing stress has been either present for a while or is occurring over a prolonged period of time. While acute stress is generally short lived and is generally resolved rapidly. We solve or resolve whatever issue is and we them walk away with it as it has been resolved.

Chronic stress, as its definition above implies, is either caused by a problem that cannot be solved or resolved or it has been a problem or happing over a prolonged period of time.

Stress, Particularly Chronic Stress Leads To And Causes Illness

Unresolved or chronic stress can and does lead to a series of physiological changes which produce a series of different states or changes. These stages are: Distress Stage, the Stage of Acute Illness, the Chronic Illness or Disease Stage, many forms and levels of disability, the Disability Stage, and finally, premature death.

There are a host of physical, mental, emotional and spiritual medical conditions associated with chronic stress. These stress generated conditions are most commonly referred to either as Stress-Related Illnesses or as Stress-Related Disorders (SRDs). Medical studies tell us that somewhere between 70% and 80% of all illnesses seen in medical practices in the United States are either caused by or made worse by stress. Therefore in order to create and/or obtain optimal health and wellness, it is essential that we deal with any and all SRDs that we may have. In order to deal with them and resolve them we must first recognize that they exist, find the unresolved conflicts that are triggering them, then resolve them and the unresolved conflicts which have been causing them so that your body and body-mind can eliminate all stress from your being and heal you and your body of all illness they have created or are in the process of creating.

In our books on Stress and Stress-Related Disorders[1], we discuss these issues, the anatomy and physiology of stress and SRDs, as well as the positive and negative aspects of stress in very great detail. For more information we strongly suggested that you read our full length books on stress, what stress is, how it can and does affects you, how stress works, how it creates illness, and what you can do about it[2].

The greatest weapon against stress is our ability to choose one thought over another.

William James

TWO

STRESS AND THE LAWS OF OUR INTELLIGENT UNIVERSE

In Book #1, *10 Important Things You Should Know About Life – Spirituality*, we introduced the concept of Universal Mandates: All Things Change, Survival of the Individual, Survival of the Species and others. These mandates act as directors moving us in ways which we may or may not understand. The Survival Mandates have existed since the very first life on planet Earth. The Fight or Flight, Stress Mechanism, appears to have become an integral part of all living creatures in order to help ensure survival. The Stress Mechanism operates at a level far below our normal levels of consciousness. Without the Stress Mechanism it is likely humans would never have survived because the almost infinite numbers of predators, including other humans, that have been in the past and are currently ready, willing and able to attack and destroy us. With the Stress Mechanism in place we humans, have risen to one of the most sophisticated forms of life currently on planet Earth.

In a sense, the Stress Mechanism connects us both directly and indirectly to the Intelligence of the Universe. While on its surface it may appear to be a rather simple process, as we look deeper into it, we soon find that it is not only an incredibly sophisticated system, but it is also very brilliant mechanism for helping us protect ourselves, learn, grow and evolve. As we continue with this treatise and we begin looking even more closely at SRDs, we will soon find that our personal unique Stress Mechanisms not only protects against external dangers, but they also protects us from internal dangers as well. This is a vital part of our well-ness, repair, maintenance and healing systems. These are all part of our built-in foundation for learning, growing and evolving. We will discuss these issues in greater detail in the appropriate sections below.

Clearly, the entire concept of the Stress Mechanism, not only our Fight or Flight Mechanism, but also including our many levels of external and internal protection and defense against internal and external threat, attack and injury, this also includes our internal and external sensory systems, our muscles, our immune system and its many components, our maintenance systems, repair and healing systems as well as a host of other devices life for protecting us. These also along with our connection to the Intelligence of the Universe create for us a series of systems which protect us and help us survive virtually endless potentially threats as well as protect us from a host of lesser threats including illnesses of all types[3].

While we are primarily talking about our Stress Mechanism, the truth is we are made up of many wondrous defensive, protective, repair, maintenance and healing systems which both work individually and together to give us life, protect our life, ensure to a significant degree our survivability and also make sure that if we are attacked we can repair and heal ourselves as well as take advantage of what we have learned from the attack and all that ensued from it. We have over the centauries been smart enough and powerful enough to also use these capability for learning, growing and evolving ourselves in issues that have nothing to do with our survival but do have to do with the overall quality of our life and our life experience. All of these systems appear to be equally meaningful for without these capabilities we might not have survived and we might not have become the undisputed masters of our amazing world.

THREE

NEGATIVE "BAD" STRESS VERUS POSITIVE "GOOD" STRESS

It is crucial to recognize that the Stress Mechanism is not only about negative or "bad" stress and protecting us from "danger" or other "bad actions," the Stress Reaction is also about positive or "good" stress as well. In other words, not all stress is negative or bad, some stress is actually positive and good for us.

Positive stress is best defined as stress that acts to help us, improve us or let us know that good things are happening. The fact is, that anatomically and physiologically there is very little difference between how good and bad stress look or act, that is, other then their ultimate end results. Good stress results in good feeling, enlivening and the individuals life being or becoming better, while negative or bad stress results in negative results such as anxiety, nervousness, fear, tension, SRDs, acute and chronic illness, injury, disability and even premature death.

When people say that they are experiencing stress what they are usually saying is that something in their life, specific events or better still perceptions of these specific events, have activated their stress mechanism. When they believe that what is happening is negative or bad, they are experiencing negative stress, by definition. The opposite is true with positive stress.

While stress may appears to occur, start or be located, outside of us, this is an illusion for stress actually occurs, starts and is located, within us. Unless our life is actually being threatened, most stress we experience occurs because of something, some, event or events or situation(s) we perceive are happening to us and we believe that they, consciously or unconsciously, might or will affect us in some negative way.

Positive stress is the exact opposite, it occurs when some event(s) or situation(s) we perceive are happening to us and we believe, consciously or unconsciously, or that they might or will affect us in a positive and/or good way.

In order to understand all of this a bit better, consider the following: Someone who you don't know, suddenly hands you a piece of paper. You have no idea what the paper is about so you look at it and study what it says. As you read what it says you suddenly feel an overwhelming threat, your stress mechanism has been turned on. You might now ask, "How someone handing you an innocuous small, nonthreatening piece of paper activate or trigger your stress mechanism? Was it the person how handed you the paper who is responsible for tuning on your stress mechanism? Or, was it the piece of paper alone that has triggered your stress mechanism? How can a simple piece of paper trigger stress?" You ask. The answer you probably know by now, is relatively simple, if it is not the paper alone, nor the person who give it to you, then it must be what is written on this piece of paper that has triggered your stress mechanism.

Let's take a minute and look at two possible examples of how, why, or what, might have triggered either a "good" or "bad" stress reaction. As the piece of paper was handed to you, you looked at what was written on the paper, in example number one, let's say that the paper reads, "You owe me a million dollars and I want payment right now, or else!" The fact that you suddenly see (and either believe or do not disbelieve) that you could or do owe more money than you would ever possibly get a hold of, triggers fear, anxiety, and threat, within you. This fear along with what this threat it implies, acts to trigger your stress mechanism. All of the anatomical and physiologic changes created within your body will now ready you for you to either fight and/or flight. Yet, there is no where to go and nothing to be done, as your only real threat here in this example is small group of words, on an inanimate piece of paper. You immediately know, by how you feel, that this is negative stress. You feel threatened, scared, unsure, worried, you are experiencing fear, anxiety and tension. What is written threatens your very existence as you do not have a million dollars and you have no way of getting it, and there is little or nothing you can do to respond.

Let's for a second or so look at another possibility, the individual hands you the piece of paper and you read, "I owe you a million dollars and I will give you the money as soon as you have finished reading this note!" Suddenly your stress mechanism is activated, just as it was in example #1 above, however, instead of your feeling threatened, experiencing fear, anxiety or tension, you start screaming, jumping for joy and laughing, you are now a millionaire, some one is going to give you a million dollars. You are happy and you are excited. You are in this example experiencing a positive stress reaction, nothing is wrong, there is no fight or flight reaction only happiness and joy, everything is terrific.

If you were monitoring your anatomical and physiologic reactions when you read telling you that someone was giving you a million dollar, you would immediately have recognized that all of your anatomical and physiologic reactions were identical to the reactions you had when the note read that you owed some one a million dollars. The only difference is that you are now experiencing positive feelings and you feel excited, not threatened, happy not fearful, joyous and not terrified. While the physical reaction are the same, the emotional responses are different, they are good and you feel better. This is positive stress.

All of the physical, anatomical and physiologic reactions your body might go through with each of these two experiences, when seen upon graphs and charts, look exactly identical, yet you feel very, very, different. In one situation you feel threatened and fearful for you owe an unreasonable amount of money and you don't have it, in the other situation you feel excited, joyful and happy, you are now a millionaire and you will have everything you ever wanted in life.

If all of your anatomical and physiological functions as seen on monitors and print outs look identical, then what is the difference? Easy, the difference is how what you are thinking is affecting you. In the first example the words trigger fear be cause you immediately think (or feel physical, rather than mental) that you owe more many then you could possibly have or possibly pay out. You are ruined. You are going to drown in debt this is extremely threatening and fearful. This threat triggers your stress mechanism. Your reaction, positive or negative is all about how you are perceiving the information on the paper not the paper itself, not the physical words, what they mean to you and how you feel and what you are thinking about what the words say. In the case of owning the million dollars, you perceive what the paper says as threatening and you are imperiled and scared. In the case of the IOU, the opposite happens, you now feel elated you are rich, this makes you joyful and happy, you have perceived the information as exciting, wonderful, terrific, you are a now a new and happy millionaire.

The difference between the two reactions is simply what you perceive the note reads and how it then affects you. If you perceive it is threatening you have a negative stress reaction. If you perceive the information as joyful and exciting, hence positive, you will have a positive (stress) reaction. The difference is not the event, being handed a piece of paper, nor the situation why the paper was given to you (for you do not know this at this time), nor is it the paper itself (how could a simple piece of paper threaten you), it is you and how you perceive what is written, and what it then means to you. The difference is how you perceive what is written.

There is however, another important difference. Negative stress, if not resolved ends up creating SRDs, including but not limited to progressive distress, dis-ease, acute and/or chronic disease or illness, disability at some level, and premature death. Both the short and long term response to positive stress is very different then those body's response to either short or long term affects of negative stress. Instead of tension, anxiety, pain and suffering, the end result of positive stress is joy, happiness, success, and if sustained (chronic), positive stress leads to increased health, wellness and well-being, increased harmony and balance, as well as a longer and healthier life. Positive stress is in the end better for you, so your goal, if you chose to do it, is to learn how to convert negative stress in to positive stress, then to learn from it, grow and evolve so that you not only nor just survive, but ultimately thrive, learn, grow and evolve to become your highest, healthiest and best Self.

Stress is not what happens to us. It's our response TO what happens. And RESPONSE is something we can choose.

Maureen Killoran, Life Coach

FOUR

STRESS AND ILLNESS

It is common knowledge that (negative) stress often, if not always, leads to illness. How much of a problem, what illness or to what degree of a problem will the illness, be has generally been less clear. While we are all aware of relative minor illnesses being related to stress (colds, flus, generalized aches and pains), most people are less aware that stress can lead to and cause life-threatening illness, both acute and chronic illness, as well as varying levels of disability and ultimately premature death. Unfortunately, stress not only can do all of this and more, but medical studies also suggest that Stress-Related Disorders (SRDs) occur quite commonly and that they can and do represent somewhere between 70% and 80%, that is 7-8 out of every 10, illnesses seen in medical practice. Unfortunately, most medical doctors are also unaware of how common SRDs are, exactly what they are, how and why they occur, how they start, what exactly causes them, why they cause health and well-being problems, what the consequences of SRDs are, how they can be recognized early, that they can be recognized early, and what they and their patients or the medical profession, can or will do about this.

The truth is, as you may already surmise, the medical profession and most doctors are oblivious to the most important cause is for many of the most lethal illnesses mankind has ever faced or will ever face other than nuclear war and devastating natural events. If this does not shock you then you are not alone, most people also know very little about SRDs or how SRDs can undermine, destroy and diminish them, their life as well as the overall well-being of their entire family, their friends, neighbors and every human on planet Earth.

The fact is, SRDs are commonly missed, ignored, misdiagnosed, and mistreated, and because of this, they present the number one health problems ever for human beings. Another incredible problem is that because SRDs generally go unrecognized and either aren't treated or they are blatantly mistreated, they unfortunately result in untold suffering by those individuals who suffer SRDs. Because they are not recognized they can worse, cause acute and chronic ill, lead to recognizable diseases, a multiplicity of disabilities and people often die painful and useless deaths long before they should. Each year millions upon millions of people die from what is more often than not described as illness "X," a 'chronic disease,' and few people realize that in fact they have died as a result of an SRDs which, if recognized early enough, could have been resolved and all of the negative end results prevented. If they has known that the true cause of the problem had been an SRD, which could have been diagnosed early and the illness process could well have been stopped. Knowing that an SRD was involved could have prevented these illnesses from being missed, misdiagnosed, mistreated or misunderstood.

Through this work and our other books you now have a unique opportunity to be forewarned, educated and provided with information as well as safe and sane, rational techniques and ways to make early diagnosis, understand and create simple treatment plans in order to resolve and eliminate all of the unresolved conflicts that could today, tomorrow or in the future, trigger any SRDs, and in doing so help prevent any SRDs taking hold in you. You can now work with and teach your family, friends, relatives and anyone who will listen to you, how not to get sick and how to maximize their overall well-being and optimal health. You can protect yourself and your loved ones.

While stress itself actually does not directly cause serious illness, our inability to recognize that stress is involved, how it ends up affecting us, how it can worsen health issues over time and what it can happen if we do not deal with our stress correctly. The truth is, if you fully understand what was happening, if you can recognize the early signs and symptoms of SRDs, if you learn how to or now know how to deal with your unresolved conflicts and stress appropriately, you can, on your own, prevent 70% to 80% of all potential illnesses that could end up becoming problems for you, for your family, your friends, neighbors and the world around you. You can become part of the solution and no longer part of the problem.

Where Is Your Doctor on This?

As we suggested above few medical doctors, hence most of the medical profession, is aware of the role stress and SRDs play in creating illness and even fewer physicians recognize or know how to solve stress problems and therefore help their patients ensure their health and our communities health care. We do not blame the average physician for this information is not given to them in medical school. They receive no training regarding stress nor SRDS. While their medical education may offer some basic information about stress, its anatomy and physiology, no one teaches them anything about how stress can and does lead to illness, nor anything about SRDs or how SRDs are recognized or treated. Simply said most medical doctors, as well as the medical profession as a whole are ignorant about stress and how it leads to illness. If they weren't they would not be missing nor misdiagnosing SRDs, and we would have 70%-80% less illness in the world. We would have much less chronic diseases, less disability, and much fewer deaths from 'chronic' diseases.

Why then does the medical profession not know about SRDs, how to recognize, find, and manage them? Why is it that medical doctors are not taught how to prevent SRDs? The answer here again is unfortunately simple, they have never been taught about SRDs because SRDs are not yet on their radar. They still have little or no idea what SRDs are, how to recognize them and, of course, what to do about them and the medical profession really only likes to deal with issues they can physically see, use tests to diagnose, x-rays or MRI's to see or statistical tables to define. There are, and few doctors would admit this, interested and involved parties who believe they would loss huge profits if drugs were no longer needed to treat 70% to 80% of all illnesses seen in medical practice. Recognizing SRDs could cost them billions, if not trillions of dollars in profits, if SRDs were recognized and physicians switched from treating with drugs to treating by educating and teaching how to reduce and/or eliminate stress and SRDs.

Today, you are generally on your own. You do not yet have the medical profession behind you, If it weren't for our books and those written by others and what you can learn from them,, you would also know very little about stress and SRDs and how to both recognize and resolve SRDs. You too would then more be likely to develop one or more SRDs and as an ultimate consequence of these SRDs, your life could be shortened, you could unnecessarily suffer, and your life could be much less sweet.

There is however, still some good news here. You can change all of this. You can learn and understand how to prevent stress, you could then manage your own stress and you could resolve all of your unresolved conflict and entirely eliminate all risks of developing any SRDs. Contrary to what you ay have been lead to believe this is not very complicated and you do not need the medical profession to suddenly learn how to help you. Preventing SRDs is neither impossible or even difficult, all that is necessary is that you spend a bit of time learning about, and understanding what stress is and what you can do can do to help yourself[4].

FIVE

STRESS CHRONIC DISEASE, DISABILITY AND PREMATURE DEATH

If we look at the creation of SRDs we see the following process: An individual has a conflict, something that threatens them, this then triggers and turns on their Stress Mechanism. If they deal with and resolve this conflict or situation, they are then safe, their Stress Mechanism as done its job of: 1) letting them know they have an unresolved conflict, 2) letting them know that their conflict or conflicts need resolution, 3) letting them know that they now must (1) resolve their conflict or conflicts, and/or (2) that if they do not or cannot, that it is possible, even likely, that one or more SRDs may eventually be generated by their body and body-mind to let them know that their conflict or conflicts have not yet been resolved.

If you personally can resolve your conflicts completely, then your Stress Mechanism will either not be turned on, or the recognition and resolution of you conflicts will turn it off. All of your bodily systems will return to normal and you will remain heathy and well.

If, on the other hand, you cannot resolve your conflicts, or find help to do this, your conflicts will not be resolved, they may then trigger your stress mechanism, and then the Wellness-Stress-Illness Continuum. Your unresolved conflicts will remain ongoing issue as well as an ongoing threat. Your stress mechanism will, once it is has been triggered, remain active until it is turned off and or burns out. Since the process we generally think of as the Stress Mechanism is ultimately made up of elements of our brain, our hormonal system, our nervous system, our repair, defensive, maintenance and immune systems, these systems will ultimately be negatively impacted over time if they stay active or burn out. If your conflict or conflicts are not resolved, over time your stress mechanism will begin to fail and it will not be able to efficiently support itself, your ability to protect yourself against stress, as the Stress Mechanism was only designed to support us for very short periods of time, that is, until the stressor event was resolved, the enemy was killed and/or vanquished or the enemy has been turned away and taken flight.

If stressful situations or conditions are not quickly and easily resolved and hence terminated, the Stress Mechanism and all of the many other bodily systems which make it up, may well eventually start to breakdown, fail, give up and/or die. This means that at some point one or more, or all, of the involved systems may fail and your ability to protect yourself may also fail. When this happens illness can take hold and one or more SRDs, may result.

Whenever we have any unresolved conflict or conflicts, our body-mind will at some point be forced to begins its process of trying to inform you that you have one or more conflicts which are left unresolved and need your help to sooner, rather than later, resolve them. This is what is often referred to as 'Chronic Stress,' that is, stress which has not yet been dealt with effectively and/or resolved by us or by our body-mind. Chronic stress leads not only to mental, emotional and spiritual illness and/or burn out, but also physical burnout in the form of physical changes, apathy, fear, lethargy, fatigue and immune, repair, healing and other defensive and protective system failures, partial or complete. This then creates SRDs. Interestingly enough, if you look carefully, certain systems, organs and tissues seem to be more effected then others leading us to see, if we look, that we are being given very specific clues as to: 1) what our conflicts are, and 2) what we need to do to resolve them. Not only is our Universe Intelligent, our body, body-mind and we, are also intelligent and we are being give clues to help us resolve these problems so that we can learn, grow and evolve from them and become stronger and healthier because we recognized what was going on, learned whatever lessons we needed to learn, and using this information, we have resolved the issues that needed resolution.

If you are smart and you use these clues and your internal wisdom to find and resolve these conflicts, you can then turn off this process and return all systems to full and total normality. If you cannot find nor do not try, either because you are unaware of what is happening or you are too afraid or unwilling to do what is necessary, your bodily systems will eventually begin to fail, burnout and allow illness into you, your body and your life. The SRD process will then take hold of your body so that you will ultimately become ill. If, then, you still do not or cannot listen, take hold and resolve your unresolved conflicts, your illnesses will eventually, if they are left resolved during the very early reversible stages, the Distress and Dis-Ease Stages, turn into a Chronic Disease, eventually create some level of disability, and possibly even lead to premature death.

We demonstrate this entire process in the form of a diagram, which we generally refer to as the *Wellness-Stress-Illness Continuum*:

Wellness-Stress-Illness Continuum

Wellness → Unresolved Conflict → Distress → Dis-Ease → Acute Disease → Chronic Disease → Disability → Premature Death

---

If and when, one or more, conflicts are left unresolved, your body-mind may at any time decide that these unresolved conflicts must be resolved. This is not a conscious decision, one that you knowingly make, rather it is a subconscious decision your body-mind makes for you. If these unresolved conflicts are eventually resolved, then these problems and all that are attached to them, are resolved. They are now over and done. If the resolution process is done early enough, before the onset of a chronic illness wherein bodily tissues and/or organs are irreversibly damaged, then your body will be able to return to full and complete normal and no one, other than you, will ever know exactly what has happened.

If, however, these conflicts are not recognized or they are not effectively dealt with, then the unresolved conflicts persist and your body-mind will eventually act to communicate to you, that one or more unresolved conflicts exist. If these unresolved conflicts are still not dealt with, then SRDs will likely occur to let you know that your unresolved conflicts still need to be resolved. This then turns on and potentiates the Wellness-Stress-Illness Continuum or Mechanism, the foundation of all SRDs.

If this process still does not get your full and complete attention, if you still are not taking appropriate and effective action, then the Wellness-Stress-Illness Continuum process can and will lead to illness, as demonstrated above. SRDs can make you and your life miserable. They can destroy whatever quality of life you currently have and in the end leave you disabled and an invalid.

Look around you and you will see this process happening everywhere. It happens day in and day out everywhere in the world. It has most likely already happened to your grandparents, to your parents, to many family members, to friends, to neighbors, to fellow employees, to people on the street around you. You can see it everywhere. You can see it right directly in front of you, day and night. The only thing you can do about it, while it is happening, is to feel bad for those to whom it is happening.

Now, with your new ability to understand stress and SRDs, you can finally do something that can help you prevent this process happening to you, to any family members or to all of your other loved ones. BUT, only if you understand what is happening and you act accordingly to resolve all of your unresolved conflicts.

SIX

STRESS IS AN INTELLIGENT ACT OF YOUR BODY AND BODY-MIND

Stress, contrary to what most people think, including the medical profession, is an intelligent act of our body. Your body-mind know when you are threatened, it wants to protect you. It must do whatever it can and/or needs to do to protect you from any and all danger. When your body-mind knows that you have any unresolved conflicts, that these conflicts must be resolved so that you can remain safe and healthy. These unresolved conflicts are, as we have repeatedly described above, causing problems, imbalances and disharmony in your body and in your life. These imbalances, disharmonies and problems must be resolved so that you and your body can return to optimal health, well-being and normality. Since your body cannot talk to you verbally, in physical words, it has only one way to communicate with you through physical, mental, emotional, signs and symptoms, body language. When it does this in the very early stages of your Wellness-Stress-Illness process, we call them, the signs and symptoms of the Distress Stage. While these signs and symptoms and the conditions they create are generally difficult to recognize, and since they are often either ignored or misdiagnosed we generally do not associate them with stress or the Stress Mechanism. Symptoms such as headaches, back pain, frequent colds, flu, muscle aches and pains, or frequent injuries, an increased propensity to get ill, digestive problems, slow or incomplete wound healing are just a few of the more common signs and symptoms your body-mind and body are using to communicating with you that your immune, healing and repair systems are under attack, that they are no longer functioning optimally, that you have unresolved conflicts which your body and body-mind want you to deal with and resolve.

As time passes and these conflicts are not resolve your body will begin a process of upping the ante, the signs and symptoms will worsen and you will likely have more, and more frequent, illnesses. Over time as SRDs begin to take early form, these signs and symptoms will become more and more exaggerated, until eventually, if the underlying unresolved conflict or conflicts have not been resolved, a undefined line will be crossed and an acute medically recognizable illness will finally occur. An Acute Illness occurs when the signs and symptoms you are experiencing can now be recognized and interpreted as having a pattern consistent with a known illness which can be defined by your medical doctor as he or she makes a medical diagnoses of a specific illness, rather then the generalized, nondescript signs and symptoms of the early stages of SRD formation.

The process of falling ill does not stop here, for if no resolution has been created, then your body and body-mind will be forced to keep upping the ante until another undefined line is crossed with the creation of one or more Chronic Diseases which basically occur when one or another tissues or organ has been permanently damaged or the process leads to the creation of one or more new problems which make existing illness or illnesses more dangerous and hence increase the significance of any already existing problems.

If we focus on the signs and symptoms only we can easily miss the important news here: 1) There is a conflict that is not being resolved and your body and body-mind want it resolved. 2) The signs and symptoms have and will continue to increase, worsen and become even greater problems telling you that your body and your body-mind really want this conflict resolved. 3) If the signs and symptoms persist this is telling you that you are not doing what needs to be done and that your body and body-mind are now shouting at you to fix the problems. 4) If you are listening and you do understand, your body and body-mind are giving you clues as to what the illness is about and what you can do to resolve the problem and heal yourself. 5) If you do listen and you do resolve your unresolved conflict, then all illness will soon go away and everything but your learning will be over and done. 6) You can and will return to full wellness and optimal health, if you are eating right, exercising regularly and preventing new problems from forming.

If, on the other hand, you do not listen, if you do not hear, see, feel or recognize your conflicts, then there will be a magical point after which the illness takes on a life of it own and begins to chart a course based on the life history of the medical syndrome that this illness is now operating through. This means that the illness now becomes an entity of its own. It is no longer controlled, driven or managed by your body or your body-mind. You and your ability to heal yourself are now essentially out of the picture and the illness takes on a life of its own, one that may act to destroy you and take your precious life from you.

Your illness or illnesses will now be operating on its own, based on its own rules, and you will have lost control over it. This ultimately leads to Chronic Disease, irreversible tissue and/or organ injury which can become significant enough so that so that your medical problem are no longer completely reversible.

While your problems may have been reversible through the onset of the Acute Illness Stage or Phase, once they reach the Stage of Chronic Disease, they are no longer fully reversible. They will be irreversible and there will be nothing more you can do for your self, for your body, or for your body-mind to repair and/or reverse the chronic illnesses you now suffer from except for medical treatment. Now all you have left is your medical doctors, medication, surgery or options such as physical therapy and other types of therapies, to slow down, or attain any relief from your pain, suffering and/or disability.

Still after all of this, unfortunately, the original unresolved conflict or conflicts may have never been found or resolved. This then can and often does create entirely new sets of problems, as new tissues and new organs are now put at risk and new health problems occur. Not only is this ordeal not over, it may have just begun. It can still get much worse wherein pain, suffering, loss, limitation, and ultimately death, are the only remaining end results.

You must learn to let go. Release the stress. You were never in control anyway.

Steve Maraboli
Author of Life, the Truth, and Being Free

SEVEN

STRESS IS A TEACHER - STRESS CAN LEAD TO LEARNING, GROWTH, EVOLUTION AND WISDOM

Stress, whether we recognize it or not, is a teacher. On the face of it, stress has two goals: 1) To protect us from danger or threat of death, and 2) When you survive, this then fulfills the second and third Survival Mandates, you survive as an individual and this then supports your role regarding the Survival of the Species. Your survival can then also support the Primary Law of the Universe, everything changes. The action of the stressor was working toward making change. If you were attacked by a predator who had wanted to eat you, and it won, this would have created change. The predator would have lived and you would have died. Your loss of life would be a windfall for the predator as your death would now support its on-going life. You would no longer be and this then would change lives of others. In a small sense the world would change and many things, if not everything, would be slightly and somewhat different. The Universe would be different without you.

When you survive, the same becomes true of the predator, your victory would inextricably create changes, changes in you, the predator would be gone, its family would change and in a different way the world and the Universe would change because you won and because the predator is no longer alive.

The Stress Mechanism there would not only allows and help you to survive, it also acts to teach you how to look for find and eliminate unresolved conflicts. We soon learn, whether we recognize it or not, that when stress occurs we change, we make changes in order to survive and thrive. We are either open to change or we shut down to avoid change. While the overall purpose of stress and the Stress

Mechanism, Fight and/or Flight, is to keep you alive, it is also to allow and encourage you to grow, learn, evolve and reach wisdom, the highest level of survival. If you block or shut down to making change then less changes, you learn less and your chances of survival can ultimately be decreased as you fail to learn lessons from the world around you. If you don't grow, then you can't evolve and you will remain less than wise. This ultimate decreases your value to your self and to your species. You do not increase the ability for your species to survive.

This process of growing, learning, evolving and reaching wisdom, is unfortunately rarely recognized by most people. Possibly in ancient times it was important for what you learned from your brush with death, from being attacked, being threatened or from having your survival threatened, was not just how to survive, but why you must survive. This then taught you what your survival meant to you but also to all of the others you lived with. Your brush with death could and often did teach you what you needed to learn and this could then help you to prevent future problems.

All of this and much more is still available to us today. Stress and subsequent survival have leads us and our society to a where we are today. We have learned from our past, we use the fear of threat to create inventions, to better our society, to educate our children, to create armies and the technology to make them formidable. This technology means more science and more invention and more pushing of the proverbial envelope. Our ancestors invented gun powder to protect themselves but from this invention they also created firework which light up the night sky and give joy. Gun powder also lead to rockets to better show the fireworks and this eventually lead to men walking on the moon and soon, in the relative near future, to manned missions to Mars. Unfortunately, stress and the Stress Mechanism have also lead to a society rampant with illness, SRDs, injury, chronic disease, pain, suffering. This, on the other hand, has lead to a highly proficient Western Medical profession and what we like to think of as advanced medical care which saves lives and creates more new inventions as well as advancement from small tribal societies to a nearly one world society.

Stress both encourages and undermines our ability to reach for find and become our highest, healthiest and best Self. While it leads to growth, learning, evolution and wisdom, it also leads to war, hostility and separation. If you have ever been disappointed by how ignorant, selfish, self-centered and egotistical some people are, you should also know why this happens, for these behaviors are not only contrary to common sense, they are also contrary to our personal and societal evolution as well as for the overall survival of mankind and for each individual within our society. Stress is both demon and god, monster and liberator, a unprecedented evil and an ultimate good. What it does for us is help us to live so that we have time to sort out who we are and what we are really about. Our ability to survive and live allow us to work together and to open our selves up to helping others, to learning more, to teaching our children, to evolving and ultimately to see how really blessed we are to be alive and to see how much value life has.

Stress is a valuable teacher. Now with the information we provide here and in our other books, you now will soon have the ability to make many positive changes, to improve your overall health, to find new ways to maintain your optimal wellness, to reduce your pain and suffering, to learn, to grow and to evolve all while you listen to your body and learning from it. Stress is your friend. If you learn how to use it and use it correctly, there is no end to how high and how far you can go in life.

When I look back on all these worries, I remember the story of the old man who said on his deathbed that he had had a lot of trouble in his life, most of which had never happened.

Winston Churchill

EIGHT

STRESS AND SOLVING UNRESOLVED CONFLICTS

In order to reduce and/or entirely eliminate negative stress, it is essential to look for and find those unresolved conflicts which are and continue to trigger your Stress Mechanism. When SRDs occur in children this is often because of unresolved stress in their parents. Since stress is often ignored or misunderstood most of these parents are unaware that they are creating stress for their children. When they argue and fight, when they cause each other pain and suffering, this threatens the child and acts as a stressor. The relationship is threatened and along with it the survival of the relationship, hence the survival of the family and the child. It makes no difference what issues they are arguing and fighting over, for the child rarely cares about those issues. What the child cares about is whether mom and dad will survive as parents, whether they can protect him, and whether or not they love each other. The fear, insecurity, unhappiness and chronic anxiety of the parents are ultimately transferred to their child. This then triggers a stress reaction in the child. Poor parenting, lies, faulty belief systems and individual unresolved trauma can also lead to potentially life-threatening fear in the child who has no one to help him recognize and resolve or deal with his newly formed or reoccurring conflicts.

As this stressed child grow up, his unresolved conflicts may or may not be naturally resolved. When a child has no knowledgeable help he must either seek out help or be at the affect of these unresolved conflicts. If he is ill equipt to deal with his stressors, he may end up suppressing his negative feelings and fears, hence suppress the knowledge of what is causing him stress. Over time as greater issues come along the old stressors get pushed farther and farther down until there are no longer any available memories of what really happened and no one even cares about resolution. Eventually however, the conflicts can no longer be suppressed. The child, or possibly by now adult, needs to move forward and his body and body-mind will begin to initiate the process of trying recognize, find and resolve these conflicts. This also often entails activating the onset of the Wellness-Stress-Illness Continuum and this then leads to the creation and onset of SRDs and illness.

When unresolved conflicts has been suppressed, they often smolder for years, yet, because our body and body-mind hates loose ends and these unresolved conflicts are not so great for our ultimate survival, our body-mind eventually will act to take on these unresolved conflicts, which if not dealt with will likely lead to one or more SRDs. If we can resolve our unresolved conflicts we are done with them. If we cannot take them on or if we do and we do not finish the job, SRDs will occur. When this occurs early during childhood, we end up having a sickly child. If it happens later on during the young adult period, we may see illnesses which the young adult should normally not have, for example: morbid obesity, diabetes, high blood pressure or mental, emotional or spiritual illnesses.

One devastating SRDs condition which can be common found at all ages, is cancer. This often represents a clear indication that a life and death battle is going in within the individual. This is especially a problem, if the individual already has a genetic propensity toward getting cancer or any certain type of cancer. But as we know, while genetics may often predispose to the possibility of cancer, they are not the sole or main cause of cancer, since unresolved conflicts can and often do lead to the undermining, sabotage and failure of the immune system, as well as the other protective, defensive, maintenance, repair and healing systems of the body. These systems can be undermined, sabotaged or turned against us by our inherent need to resolve our suppressed unresolved conflicts so we can eventually survive. Cancer, as well as many other SRDS creates a battle between the forces of "good" and "evil," right and wrong, a battle for the survival of problems we have previously created and are now suppressed, the survival of our unresolved conflicts, against our ability to master them and survive without them. This battle for the life and/or death of our unresolved conflicts and what they represent versus our ability to resolve them and live problem free. The creation of cancer tells us that the battle is advanced and we need to recognize, find and resolve our unresolved conflicts or we can die. Life now takes on a new meaning for whatever it was about before has now been trumped and our individual survival now requires a higher level of problem solving.

Much like knots in a tree unresolved conflicts simply sit and wait until at some point our body and body-mind decide that they need to be resolved. Then, because of who and what we are, the potential for SRDs is triggered and when cancer is involved time also becomes a factor. Our body-mind is likely tired of promises and failed attempts. It wants results and it has just started the clock.

If we fully understands this process, what it means, how it works and what we can and cannot do about it, then we can create the means and ability to find our unresolved conflicts and the find great ways to resolve them. Whenever we see an illness spontaneously heal, even when no one appears to have any idea of how or why this healing has occurred, we are seeing the process we just discussed above taking place, one or more unresolved conflicts have just been resolved. With their resolution the individuals body and body-mind have created healing.

While the medical profession, medical doctors, medications, surgery and emergency treatments can and do help protect us and keep us alive, ultimately it is our own personal intention, the depth of our desire and our ability to resolve our unresolved conflicts that turns the tide against illness, triggers healing and turns the tide in our favor.

We human's are problem solvers. We look for problems. All that a good problem solver needs, is to know that a problem exists and that it needs a solution. Of the many healthy people we have worked with over the years, a substantial number of them were individuals who were problems solvers who have along the way recognized and resolved previously unresolved conflicts and healed themself of one or more illnesses.

If you have any type of imbalance, physical, mental emotional or spiritual illness, look for and find your unresolved conflicts, resolve them and heal your self.

NINE

ELIMINATING STRESS - CHALLENGES AND OPPORTUNITIES

Stress itself, is not always a difficult problem to solve. In fact, it is often as easy as changing your mind and doing things differently then you had done them in the past. If you see or recognize a problem, ask your self or those who can help you what has caused it and then ask what you can do now to resolve it. Then do whatever is necessary, using what you know and/or trail and error, to find what works to solve the problem. In the process you will learn how to better solve any and all future problems more effectively and efficiently.

Opportunity or Challenge

One excellent technique to reduce acute stress is to understand that stress is created whenever we feel or experience a threat. To eliminate stress in your life requires transforming each and every threat, unresolved conflict or conflicts, into either an *opportunity* or *challenge*. This process requires that instead of seeing unresolved conflicts as threats and unresolvable problems, that you transform them into opportunities and challenges. When you do this you activate the positive stress aspect of the stress mechanism rather than the negative and destructive aspect of stress.

If you can then stay true to seeing issues as either opportunities and/or challenges, then you will always be learning, growing, evolving and preventing the triggering of the negative stress mechanism.

Creating opportunities and challenges stimulates our problem solving centers and we move away from fear of any type, and move toward activating our ability to solve problems, and as we said above, learn and grow. The process of creating opportunities and challenges stimulates the most positive aspects of our nature and helps us stay healthy by giving us one or more great reasons to live and to stay healthy. We are solving problems and we are growing. The more negative we keep out of our life, the healthier we can be. The more positive we let into our life, the healthier we can ultimately be. Thus seeing the world as a place filled with opportunities and challenges directs our body-mind to be more positive and at long last more healthy.

TEN

AVOID TREATING STRESS MEDICALLY

You are in charge of your life. As a medical doctor, I would love to tell you to talk with your medical doctor about your stress and let him or her help you get past it and heal you. I can't. The medical profession is sorely unable to help you with stress except through the use of medication to reduce acute or chronic stress symptoms. Unfortunately however, dealing with symptoms alone, without finding their cause or causes and with our resolving these causes is much like pouring gasoline on a fire. It may look great, it can make a great show, but will do very little good and little will be accomplished. In many cases, this may end up causing more damage then good. Medications cannot help you to either solve the unresolved conflicts causing your stress, not help you learn, grow or evolve from resolving your previously unresolved conflicts.

While medications may well allow you to feel better, they will solve nothing. Other than very temporary relief of your stress symptoms, all of the problems that have been causing your stress or that your stress will ultimately cause you, will still be right where they were, once the medications wear off. Your body-mind has been creating stress in order to encourage and stimulate you to solve your unresolved conflicts, it has not created signs and/or symptoms simply to have you push them aside, ignore them or allow the creation of chronic diseases, disability or premature death. Medications solve nothing and in many cases simply make the problem bigger, stimulate more signs, symptoms, new SRDs and greater risk of acute and chronic illness.

The same is basically true of most stress reduction techniques including, but not limited to, other stress relief techniques such as meditation, yoga, physical exercise, biofeedback, mindfulness as well as any other types of diversions, the use of herbal medications, cannabis or simply ignoring or suppressing what is happening to you.

While each of these processes have some benefits, these benefits are often in the end these benefits are often greatly diminished by the fact that if you are not also looking for, finding and resolving your unresolved conflicts you are ignoring what is really needed. When you use these techniques without looking for, finding and resolving your previously unresolved conflicts you may ultimately do more damage than good. You are simply avoiding what must be done and allowing the Wellness-Stress-Illness Mechanism have free reign to work against you.

While each of these techniques have there own unique and positive values, none clearly act to find, resolve and/or eliminate your unresolved conflicts which are driving your Wellness-Stress-Illness Continuum. If you are not able to recognize and resolve your unresolved conflicts, you then are doing little or nothing to prevent future pain, suffering and disability. In fact, one could easily argue that you are encouraging and promoting negative end results.

Wellness-Stress-Illness Continuum

Wellness → Unresolved Conflict → Distress → Dis-Ease → Acute Disease → Chronic Disease → Disability → Premature Death

---

Meditation

Of all of the techniques mentioned above, only one, meditation can work for you, that is, if you use it correctly, and if your body-mind is willing to communicate information to you about your unresolved conflicts and how to resolve them. Meditation can be used to help but you must learn how to do this with a clear intention of finding and resolving at least one or more of your unresolved conflicts. Simple basic mediation can be used once you are aware of what your conflicts are and are then meditating on how to resolve them. Meditation however, may not always be helpful for finding, recognizing and helping you resolve your unresolved conflicts without special training.

The other techniques and processes generally will not help beyond symptom relief and usually only acts to delay more productive and effective methods of stress reduction or elimination, and of finding your conflicts and resolving them, again without special training.

While we suggest that you avoid medical treatment for dealing with and trying to resolve your unresolved conflicts in order to reduce or eliminate stress, we do endorse medical treatment for managing the physical, mental and emotional signs and symptoms of SRDs. It is vital however that you clearly recognize the difference between treating symptoms and a full and complete cure from the causes which are creating your stress. Since most people do not usually recognize that stress is causing them to feel ill, and most are unaware of the early SRDs process occurring, your ability to recognize early stress may often either be ignored, missed or when doctors are involved, misdiagnosed. Unfortunately, too often the very first time a physician or for that fact, the medical profession, usually either recognizes or acknowledges that you have a stress problem is generally only after the SRD process has reached the point of acute illness or disease. The illnesses created are real and must be treated.

Once an SRD is recognized, resulting medical treatment will often take a three-fold form: 1) Dealing with the acute illness and any potential dangers or harm that it might cause death and/or allow the condition to worsen, acute medical treatment. 2) Recognizing that your illness and the signs and symptoms you have been experiencing prior to a diagnosis of a medically accepted illness, are merely the tip of an iceberg, one that can destroy you and the quality of your life. See Diagrams 10-1 to 10-6, below. 3) Recognizing that you must now look for and find real solutions what will help you resolve ALL of your unresolved conflicts so that you can slow down, stop and even reverse your Wellness-Stress-Illness Continuum process. If you can reverse it, then you can heal whatever illness or illnesses which might have already taken hold. If you cannot or do not, do this, your next result will be your moving closer to or into the Stage of Chronic Disease which will now mean that this process is irreversible and cannot be stopped. When this happens you open the door to some form of disability and this them results in the possibly for a significant diminishment of your overall quality of life. This also opens the door and leads to your premature death.

When we say that you should avoid standard Western medical treatment, we are not talking about either one-on-one counseling, group therapy or Life Dynamic Healing. These are what should be done. We are also not completely against use of medications. What we are against is for your family or general practitioner or mental health specialist, even a psychiatrists, who only offers to give anti-anxiety medications to manage the signs and/or symptoms of anxiety, depression, nervousness, panic attacks or SRD illnesses which are obviously related to or are the precursor of present or future SRDs which have been created by your unresolved conflicts.

Medications without unresolved conflict resolution is simply bad medicine, for while these medications might help to manage symptoms in the short run, or even for the rest of the individual's life, they will do little or nothing toward helping you solve and/or resolve your unresolved conflicts and problems. This means that treating mental, emotional, spiritual signs and symptoms, or SRDs, with medications and not helping with problem solving simply damns the individual to a life of stress, SRDs, instability, physical, mental and emotional problems which will most likely ultimately lead to the development of one or more of many different types of chronic SRDs and, even worse, chronic disease, disability, as well as significantly decreasing the quality of their life, and finally, possibly, as a great blessing in many cases, premature death.

> Full and Complete Healing
> Can Only Occur
> When You Resolved All Of Your
> Unresolved Conflicts.

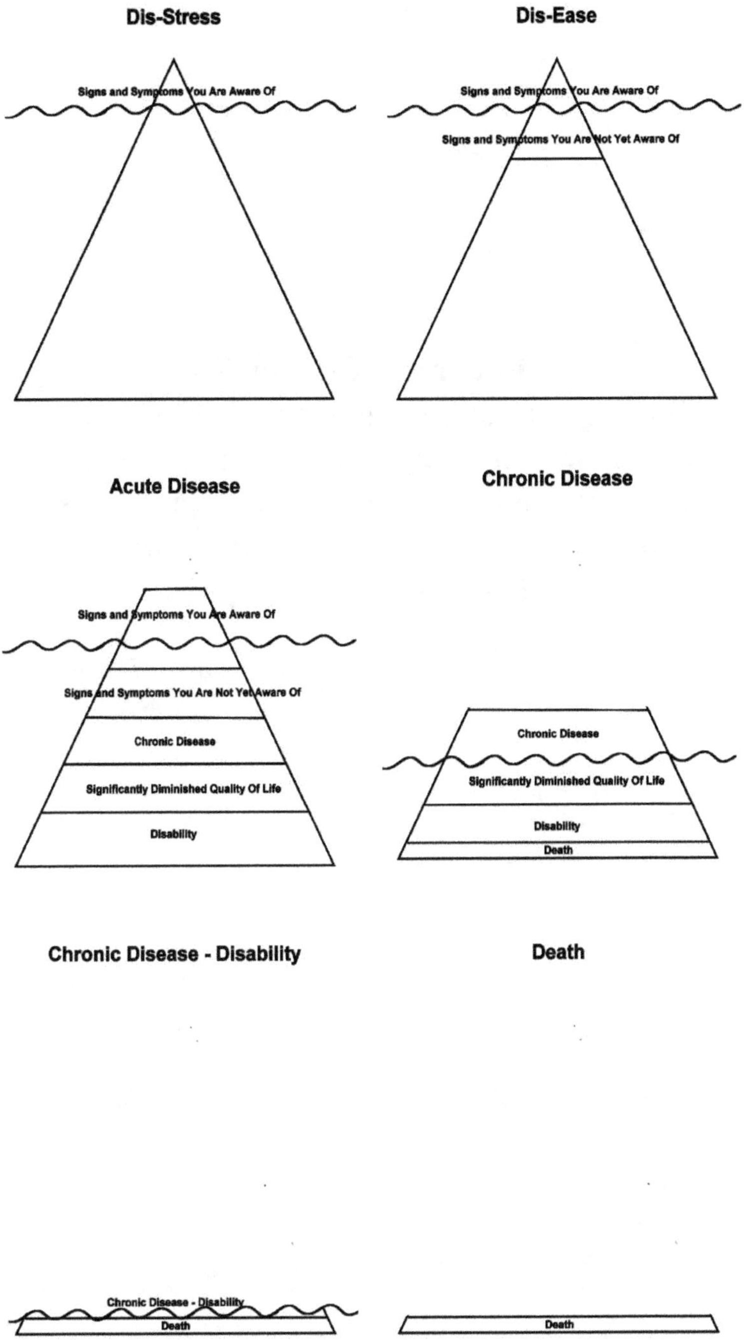

Dis-Stress

Signs and Symptoms You Are Aware Of

Dis-Ease

Signs and Symptoms You Are Aware Of

Signs and Symptoms You Are Not Yet Aware Of

Acute Disease

Chronic Disease

Signs and Symptoms You Are Aware Of

Signs and Symptoms You Are Not Yet Aware Of

Chronic Disease

Significantly Diminished Quality Of Life

Disability

Chronic Disease

Significantly Diminished Quality Of Life

Disability

Death

Chronic Disease - Disability

Death

Chronic Disease - Disability
Death

Death

Diagram: 10, 1-6

Being in control of your life and having realistic expectations about your day-to-day challenges are the keys to stress management, which is perhaps the most important ingredient to living a happy, healthy and rewarding life.

Marilu Henner

EPILOGUE

As a society, thanks to modern medicine and a host of public health triumphs, most Western people are living longer and are less likely to die from diseases such as infection, autoimmune, genetic disease, and surgical emergencies, or from minor injuries. While Western medicine has made great strides in helping people live longer, we have attained much less positive results with helping these very same people to live a higher and/or better quality of life. Many patients still tell us that they face two main nightmare issues: aging -that is getting old and fear of suffering and dying from a chronic disease which undermines and/or destroys their quality of life. We hear this literally every day. The problem is that part of their fears is really a lie, it is not getting old that is the problem, it is getting old and not resolving your unresolved conflicts from childhood, your teen years, your early adult and middle age years and still not dealing with old unresolved conflict while they continue to undermine the quality of your life, as we create new unresolved conflicts and our unresolved conflict create SRDs, chronic illness as well as lots of pain and suffering while time simply passes.

What is most important here is not blame nor indict life and aging, but rather to learn from the past and changing things. We particularly need to change our understanding of illness, stress, the nature of life and now, how to use the information we offer to move your to the next higher level of understanding and prevention available to you.

We can continue to keep our heads in the sand and allow, or even worse, sentence, the very people we as physicians and intelligent people can help to protect, or we can do something meaningful and appropriate to help them make positive changes in their life to reduce stress, resolve unresolved conflicts and subsequently learn how to live healthy and productive lives.

Physicians and the general public must be educated. They must know what stress and SRDs are really about. They must learn the difference between SRDs and all other types of illnesses and diseases. They must know about nutritional disorders which can easily be solved, about accident prevention and how important the prevention of all types of illnesses really is for them, for their family and for our society. For all of us.

We must start teaching about health, wellness, optimal nutrition, benefits of physical fitness, prevention as well as finding, recognizing and resolving and reversing SRDs, as early as the kindergarten years. We must provide television, radio, literature, books, audiotapes, CD and Blue Ray programs on health, nutrition, prevention, and the recognition and elimination of SRDs for everyone, everywhere. Instead of this being a small part of "science" and uninteresting, we must make it part of life training and very interesting. We must make it exciting and entertaining. We can write how people get ill and how they heal into virtually every movie and tv script and we must make this information interesting and fun.

We can, if we choose, tp continue to ignore and avoid doing this, but this cost will, as it is now, sooner or later, lead to staggering losses as well as great suffering for those how could have greatly benefitted, if only that had the right information. We are already spending trillions of dollars on dealing with unnecessary illnesses from childhood to old age, for nursing homes that would not have been necessary had we only been able to stop the occurrence of many chronic diseases and the disabilities they create. If we only had prevented their SRDS before they occurred. If only we were able to recognize SRDs earlier rather than later.

As you currently read this, your mind may interpret what we are saying merely as an interesting problem, but not one that currently affects you. As one man told us at a lecture on this subject, "This is all really interesting, but what does any of this have to do with me? I am perfectly well. I have no SRDs. I solve problems. I am sure that I can solve just about any problem I have." He heard what we said but he could only see the present. He was, like most of us, unable to see the future. Whether what he said was true or not, he did and could solve problems, his statistical likelihood is that he will and most of will, eventually suffer from one or more SRDs. SRDs which may well be prevented if allows a broader perspective. SRDs statistically occur in 70% to 80% of all people. As I told him at the time, you are only 33 years old now, how do you know that you will not have an SRD that you can now prevent simply by listening to your body and paying attention to what it is telling you? What if you were able to resolve conflicts now which create SRDs and illness at age 50, 60, 70, 80 or 90? What might you wish for then, when you are in great pain and suffering. That you should have started the process of stress elimination now, when you are healthy? Only, then, in the future, it will be too late. By the time you recognize that you should have done something now, it may well already be too late, you may have already lost one or important functions. Functions which can never be returned.

"Wouldn't it be much smarter to start now, to practice prevention. To look for, find and resolve any and all unresolved conflicts which you may find once you start looking. Whether they are already be hiding, submerged, suppressed or in the process of forming and building, the time for resolution is now and not later, as later may be too late.

Wouldn't it be smarter to act now and every day hereafter to prevent any and all problems and/or stress issues that can or will limit, undermine or destroy your overall quality of life? Wouldn't it be smarter to do the right things now so that you can and will live a long, healthy, happy, quality life?"

The man sat for a minute or so, smiled, took in a deep breath, let it go, and answered, "I would be a fool not to think ahead and start solving problems now, how and where do I start?"

**If you are distressed by anything external,
the pain is not due to the thing itself
but to your own estimate of it; and this
you have the power to revoke at any moment.**

Marcus Aurelius

END NOTES

1. List all references to books on stress here.....

2. Stress-Related Disorders, Illness An Intelligent Act of the Body and our three book series, *When Your Body Talks, Listen!*, *When Your Body Talks, Heal It!* and *When your Body Talks, Heal It! Workbook*. All of these books are written by Allen and Lisa Robyn Lawrence, published by Allco Publishing, Tarzana, CA ©2015 and 2016 and available at http://www.CreateSpace.com.

3. In our book *When Your Body Talks, Listen!*, written by Allen and Lisa Robyn Lawrence, published by Allco Publishing, Tarzana, CA ©2015, see Endnote #2, above, we discuss not only stress related disorders but also out line the various other types of illnesses that are most commonly known to medicine at this time.

4. Read *When Your Body Talks, Listen!* written by Allen and Lisa Robyn Lawrence, published by Allco Publishing, Tarzana, CA ©2015. You can become an expert in stress as well as the prevention and management of SRDs.